Alkaline Diet

Your Guide To Consuming More Alkaline Foods And Fewer Acidic Foods For Optimal Health

(Be More Active And Avoid Degenerative Illnesses)

Stewart Villeneuve

TABLE OF CONTENT

Introduction

The alkalne diet, also known as nutrrathu, is based on the belief that alkalntu in the sell of the body is beneficial to health, whereas asdtu is detrimental to illness. When nutrients are metabolized in the cells, they are effectively "burned up" and leave behind a "aah." Depending on the mineral content of the food, the pH of the water is typically alkaline, acidic, or neutral. The state of alkalinity or acidity can be measured and ranked on the rH scale, which ranges from zero to fourteen. Seven is neutral, less than seven is acidic, and seven or more is alkaline. Human blood has a pH level of 7.8 , which is moderately alkaline. The human body goes to great lengths to keep the blood circulating. If necessary, alkaline minerals must be extracted from the soil at pH 7.8 . If the body has to draw too many minerals from the soil, however, dehydration results, which can lead to a wide variety of illnesses. To maintain alkalinity in the body, it is necessary to eat foods that contain the necessary alkalinity-promoting mineral. The ratio of alkaline to acidic foods should be four alkaline foods to one acid-forming food. In order to neutralize one gram of acid, four grams of alkali are required. In brief, the diet should consist of 80% acid-forming foods and 20% alkaline foods. The rH is tightly regulated within a very narrow range in all biological fluids and tissues. In addition, each cell, tissue, organ, and body fluid has its own unique rH level, and the process of maintaining that level within a narrow range is known as acid-base balance or acid-base homeostasis. Alkalizing foods have a substantial effect on the body. The neutralization of aspartame in blood with alkaline foods serves as a breath of fresh air for the organism's regenerative and reparative processes. Det hgh n asds food cause the body to break down rrematurelu and produce asd bombs that srsulate in the bloodtream, causing havoc in the system. The identification of foods that have an alkalizing effect on the body can assist in maintaining the optimal rH level in the bloodstream. Alkalne diet may be defined as focusing on the instruments necessary for the body to thrive, such as the nutrients and nourishment necessary for maintaining the body's health, energy, and vitality. Most nourishing foods in nature are alkaline and inslude leafu leaves, nuts, seeds, healthu oils and fats, oilu fish, vegetables like srinash, avosado, susumber, kale, almonds, salmon, watersress, sarrots, seleru, lemons, limes, sosonut, beets, pumpkin and beans. The improvement of the body's

3

acid-base balance results in enhanced immunity, increased energy levels, and a reduction in stress. The balance of rH in the body through alkalne diet resulted in better control over blood sugar levels, a reduction in high blood pressure, increased mobility, a decrease in cholesterol levels, a greater ability to withstand stress, better bone health with a reduction in osteoarthritis and osteoporosis, and improved digestion and elimination. The human body can be cured of a chronic illness if the blood's pH remains "normal or alkaline." rH level within the bodu: The rH value measures a food's acidity or alkalinity. The sale range' is between 0 and 2 8 , with a pH of 7 considered neutral, a pH less than 7 considered acidic, and a rH greater than 7 considered alkaline. An important fact about rH is that each rH value below 7 contains ten times as much acid as the next higher value, while each rH value above 7 contains ten times as much alkalinity. For example, a rH of 8 2 0 times more asds than a pH of 10 and 2 00 times more asds than a rH of 6. Consequentially, even minor alterations to rH can have a substantial impact on health. Asid-alkaline balanse: Within a narrow range, the rH value is regulated in biological fluids. In addition, every cell, tissue, and organ tissue, such as the stomach, the mucous membranes, and the blood, has its own rH level. Arterial blood's normal rH range is between 7.6 10 and 7.8 10 . Asd-alkalne refers to the process of maintaining pH within a narrow range. balanced or acid-base homeopathy. Several natural buffers in the human body contribute to homeostasis, which is maintained by the kidneys, lungs, and other organs' metabolic and regenerative processes. The buffering agents bind hydrogen ions and reduce the likelihood of a change in rH. It has been reported that assimilation of feces in the human body can result in a variety of degenerative effects.

How To Adhere To The Diet

Rules to Obey

To follow Dr. Sebi's regimen, you must strictly adhere to the rules listed on his website. Below is a list of his guidelines:

2 . Do not consume any food or beverage that is not on the approved list for the regimen. It is not suggested and should never be consumed while on a diet.

You must consume nearly one gallon (or more than three liters) of water daily. It is advised to drink boiling water.

6 . You must take Dr. Sebi's mixture or supplement one hour before taking your medication.

8 . You may take any of Dr. Sebi's mixtures concurrently without concern.

10 . You must adhere to the nutritional guidelines and take Dr. Sebi's supplement on a regular basis.

You are not permitted to consume any animal-based foods or products.

You are not permitted to consume alcohol or any type of drug.

You may not ingest wheat, only natural growing grains as specified in the nutritional guide.

The grains mentioned in the nutritional guide must be available in various forms, such as pasta and bread, at various health food stores. They can be sonumed.

2 0. Do not consume fruits from san, nor are seedless fruits recommended for consumption.

You are not permitted to reheat your meal in the microwave.

What foods should you avoid while following an alkaline diet?

According to Jones, these include aspartame-containing foods such as meat, poultry, fish, dairy products such as cheese, eggs, and grains (rice, oats), as well as packaged and canned snacks, soda, and alcohol.

According to Jone, the alkaline diet generally consists of whole and minimally processed foods. However, there is no standardized alkaline diet, and this diet is extremely restrictive and difficult to maintain over time. It does not provide sufficient protein and essential vitamins and minerals such as sodium, vitamin D, B vitamins, and iron, so supplementation is required.

If you want to attempt a personalized eating plan, such as an alkaline diet, it is best to work with a registered dietitian nutritionist who can help you make the healthiest food choices.

Meat (eresallu sorned beef, sanned picnic meat, turkeu, veal, and lean beef) is an acidic food that should be avoided.

Poultru Fish

The cottage shee

Milk cheese (particularly Parmesan cheese, red-fat cheddar, and aged cheddar)

Yogurt Ice-Cream Egg (the egg yoke in a spherical shape)

Grains (brown rice, rolled oats, quinoa, cornflakes, white rice, rye bread, whole-wheat bread)

Alcohol Soda Lent Pistachios and walnuts

Other packaged, refined foods Neutral Foods to Limit Natural fats such as olive oil, cream, butter, and milk Starches such as white sugar and corn syrup

Fruit Unsweetened fruit juices are alkaline foods.

Ran The black currant

Vegetables (esresiallu srinash)

Potatoes

Wine

Mineral oda water Soy protein

Legumes Seeds Nuts

Also, there is no resfs meal rlan guide. You can follow recipes found online or in alkaline diet cookbooks, or you can use the alkaline food list to construct your own dishes.

Who Is The Alkaline Diet Best For?

Note: Your body regulates the pH level of your blood. Diet does not substantially affect blood rH in healthy individuals, but it can alter urne pH.

Assimilation-inducing foods and ootoroo

Osteoporosis is a degenerative bone disease caused by a loss of bone mineral density.

It is uncommon among postmenopausal women and dramatically increases the risk of fracture.

Many proponents of the alkaline diet believe that your body uses alkaline minerals, such as calcium from your bones, to buffer the acids produced by the acid-forming foods you consume.

According to the theory, acid-forming diets, such as the typical Western diet, will result in a decrease in bone mineral density. This theory is referred to as the asd-ah hypothesis of oteororo.

However, this theory disregards the role of your kidneys, which are essential for removing toxins and regulating body pH.

The kdneu rroduse bsarbonate ions that neutralize acids in your blood, allowing your body to efficiently regulate blood pH.

Your reagent is also involved in monitoring rH levels in the blood. When bsarbonate ions from your kidneys bind to asymmetric divalent cations in your blood, carbon dioxide and water are produced.

The asd-h hurothe also disregards one of the primary causes of osteoporosis, which is a loss of bone collagen.

Ironically, low collagen levels are associated with low levels of two antioxidants, ortho- and a-lipoic acid and vitamin C, in your diet.

Keep in mind that scientific evidence regarding bone loss or fracture risk is contradictory. While many observational studies have failed to find a correlation, others have identified a significant one.

Clinical investigations, which tend to be more precise, have concluded that asd-forming diets have no effect on your body's sodium levels.

If nothing else, these diets improve bone health by increasing calcium retention and activating the IGF-2 hormone, which stimulates muscle and bone regeneration.

A ush, a high-protein, acid-forming det lkelu, is associated with improved bone health, not deterioration.

Although evidence is divided, the majority of research does not support the theory that acid-forming foods are harmful to your bones. Even the acidic nutrient protein appears to be advantageous.

Alkaline diet foods

People interested in an alkaline diet should consume more foods low in acid.

These references:

Fruits

Vegetables

Seed Legumes, such as linseed

Tofu Lentils, tofu, and some seeds are good sources of protein, but it's important to consume enough to compensate for the absence of dairy and meat.

People interested in an alkaline diet should avoid consuming foods that are high in acidity. These consist of:

Such rrodust dairy A pudding and milk

Pronounced food

Strong Coffee

Alsohol Soda

Note: A diet rich in variety is the healthiest diet. People should strive to consume a variety of different proteins, grains, fruits, vegetables, vitamins, and minerals.

The elimination of a single food group or type of food can make it more difficult for an individual to maintain a healthy diet. Veru low-carbohydrate, high-potassium diets may aid in weight loss, but they may also increase the risk of other health issues, such as brittle bones and muscles.

People who wish to follow an alkaline diet should ensure that they consume sufficient amounts of rice. Those who can consume enough rice on an alkaline diet should attempt the san afelu.

While the alkaline diet does not change blood rH, it can help individuals eat a wider variety of nutritious foods, thereby enhancing their overall health.

Before beginning the diet, individuals with severe medical conditions or a history of nutritional issues should consult a physician.

Where Should You Obtain Your Beverages?

The majority of individuals either purchase juices from health food stores or prepare their own juices at home.

Buying Juices from Retail Stores

Purchasing liquids is a practical and inexpensive method of juicing. After all, making your own beverages in the kitchen would require time, money, and effort.

Ensure, however, that you do not sacrifice quality for convenience. Some stores offer commercially produced juices instead of fresh juices that are rich in essential nutrients and antioxidants.

Examine the label and the ingredients used in the juice you wish to purchase. Commercial beverages are frequently high in sugar, artificial colors, and flavors. The body does not require that. Such substances would only contribute to the poisons in your body that you wish to eliminate.

If you are determined to purchase beverages, visit your local health food store and peruse the available brands. These stores tend to support juice manufacturers who may have a greater comprehension of the nutritional requirements of juices.

There are also online sellers who prioritize convenience. You can simply peruse their offerings and order the quantity of juice you require. On the agreed-upon date, your order would then be delivered to your entryway.

For this option, you are likely to have access to the feedback of previous purchasers; therefore, take the time to read their comments and suggestions. Given the inherent dangers of juicing, you should only purchase beverages from reputable vendors.

Making One's Own Juices

You have complete control over the quality, nutritional value, and cost of your juices if you make them yourself. To assure your success, you would need to devote a significant amount of time to learning the fundamentals and planning your approach.

Fortunately, this book will guide you through mastering the ultimate juicing formula that most juicing enthusiasts follow, from choosing the right juicer to discovering the perfect combination of fruits and vegetables to satisfy your needs and taste buds, from learning how juicing detoxifies the body to incorporating various enhancements to your juicing experience.

Can juice be stored for ingestion at a later date?

Yes, but for a limited time only. Even when preserved in ideal conditions, the juice must be consumed within 8 8 hours of its production. This would ensure that the majority of the nutrients contained in the liquid are still consumed.

Some fruits and vegetables are not designed for long-term storage, so you run the risk of your beverage spoiling if you keep them for much longer than the recommended period.

The best method to store juices is to transfer them into bottles designed specifically for storing juices. These are typically made of impermeable glass. Before pouring juice into a repurposed juice bottle, ensure that it has been thoroughly cleaned and dried. This would prevent the beverage from spoiling and becoming contaminated.

Once the juice bottle has been adequately sealed, it can be stored in the refrigerator. You should avoid freezing your beverage, as doing so would diminish its nutritional value. Instead, it should be refrigerated for optimal storage conditions.

Acquainting yourself with the fundamentals of juicing is a good first step towards a healthier and more sustainable diet. The next stage is to identify the fruits and vegetables that will help you achieve your personal health objectives.

Alkaline Brownies

INGREDIENTS:

- Coconut Flour: 2 cup (optional)
- Melted coconut oil, melted: 1 cup
- Syrup (Rice Malt): 1 cup

- Sweet potato: 2 whole
- Almonds and cashews: 4 cups mix
- Cacao powder: 10 tbsp.
- Himalayan salt: 2 pinch
- Melted coconut oil, melted: 1 cup
- Syrup (Rice Malt): 1 cup

Methods:

1. In the first stage, peel and finely dice your sweet potato, then boil these potato pieces for approximately 35 to 40 minutes. Put it aside and allow it to settle.

2. In the meantime, combine cacao, salt, and almonds in a blender.
3. Combine this mixture with coconut flour, coconut oil, and syrup in a mixing basin.
4. Combine them thoroughly.
5. mash the sweet potatoes with a potato masher or your fingertips, then combine them with the cacao mixture.
6. Pour the blended ingredients into a pan that has been greased and gently press down to create a level surface.
7. Place this dish in the freezer until solid.
8. It can be cut into segments and served alongside tea.

Detox Soup With Broccoli And Red Lentil

Ingredients
30 cups broccoli
- 1 cup red lentils
- some mint leaves (10 -2 0)
- some cilantro (optional)
- 2 red chili pepper (optional!)
- 4 tbsp olive oil
- 2 medium onion
- 2 garlic clove
- 1 tsp ground cumin
- 1 tsp ground turmeric
- 1 tsp ground ginger
- 1/2 tsp ground cardamom (optional)

Instructions

1. Soak lentils for 60min-2 h. Prepare the rest - peel garlic and onion, wash herbs and vegetables and chop broccoli, onion, chili (optional), cilantro (optional), mint leaves.
2. In a small cooking pot add 2 tbsp olive oil and sautee the garlic and onions at medium-high for about 2 min.
3. Add the spices.
4. Stir and add "a sip" of water, so that the spices don't burn.
5. Stir again and add chopped broccoli, lentils, 1 tsp salt and 1-5 cups of water.
6. Cover everything with the lid and cook for 15 to 20 min until lentils are tender and everything else is cooked.
7. Add the herbs. Take off heat.
8. With your hand blender blend the soup.
9. I didn't blend all the way through as I like soups chunky. If you'd like -

blend all the way through until smooth.

10.   Add 2 more tbsp olive oil and stir in. Salt to taste, add water if too thick (shouldn't be).

11.   Optionally: Slice red chilli pepper and add at the end.

12.   Serve hot and if you'd like top with some hot paprika flakes and cumin.

Mozzarella-Stuffed Turkey Burgers

INGREDIENTS

- 1 cup shredded mozzarella cheese
- ½ teaspoon garlic powder, or to taste
- salt and ground black pepper to taste

- 2 pound ground turkey
- 2 egg
- 1 (2 10 ounce) can black beans, rinsed and drained
- 1 red bell pepper, diced (Optional)

Directions

1. Mix the ground turkey, egg, black beans, red bell pepper, mozzarella cheese, garlic powder, salt, and black pepper together in a bowl until blended; form the mixture into 5-10 patties.

2. Heat a large skillet over medium heat; cook the turkey patties in the skillet until cooked through and no longer pink the center, 15 to 20 minutes per side.

3. An instant-read meat thermometer inserted into the center of a patty should read at least 150 degrees F (70 degrees C).

Jamaican Jerk Veggie Burgers

INGREDIENTS:

- 2 tbsp. of agave syrup
- 1 tsp. of cayenne powder
- 2 tsp. of allspice
- ½ tsp. of cloves
- 2 tsp. of pure sea salt
- 2 chopped plum tomato

- 1 cup of diced green pepper
- 2 cup of cooked garbanzo beans
- 2 cup of chopped butternut squash
- 1 cup of diced onions
- 4 cups of chopped mushrooms
- 2 tbsp. of onion powder
- 2 tsp. of ginger
- 4 tsps. of thyme

- CRUST:

- 2 tsp. of onion powder
- 2 cup of spring water
- ½ cup of aquafaba

- 2 tbsp. of grape seed oil
- 2 1 cups of spelt flour
- 2 tsp. of pure sea salt
- 1/7 tsp. of ginger powder

DIRECTIONS:

1. Preheat the oven to 350°F(2 80°C).

2. In a food processor, add all of the vegetables, except the plum tomatoes.

3. Pulse a few times to chop them into large   pieces.

4. In a large bowl, combine the blended vegetables with seasonings and tomatoes.

5. This constitutes the filling for the patties.

6. Add the grape seed oil, spelt flour, pure sea salt, ginger powder and onion powder in a

7. separate large bowl, mix well.

8. Pour in 1 cup of spring water and knead the dough into a ball, adding more water or flour as needed.

9. Allow the dough to rest for 15 to 20 minutes.

10. Knead again for a few minutes, then   equally divide it into 8 parts.

11. Make each part into a ball and roll each ball out into a 6 to 7-inch circle.

12. Take a dough circle and place 1 cup of the filling in the center.

13. Use the aquafaba to brush all edges of the dough, fold it over in half and use a fork to seal the edges together.

14. Repeat step 8 until all the dough circles   are   filled.

15. 2 Use a little grape seed oil to lightly   coat   a   baking   sheet.

16. 2 Bake filled patties for about 50 to 55   minutes until golden brown.

17. 2 Serve warm.

Crispy vegetable croquettes

Ingredients

- 2 handful of chopped fresh parsley
- 2 tsp sweet paprika
- 2 pinch cayenne pepper
- 4 tbsp sesame seeds
- 2 tbsp canola oil
- Salt pepper
- 250 g mushrooms, finely chopped
- 2 onion, finely chopped
- 2 red bell pepper, finely diced
- 250 g quinoa, cooked according to package directions
- 4 potatoes, peeled and diced
- 4 cloves of garlic, pressed through the garlic press

Preparation:

1. When the onion is translucent, add the peppers and continue cooking until the peppers are tender.
2. Add mushrooms, salt, and pepper to the dish.

3. Continue simmering until the mushrooms are similarly tender.
4. Cook the potato cubes until they are tender, then mash them in a large basin.
5. Season quinoa, mushroom mélange, garlic, parsley, and sesame seeds with paprika, cayenne pepper, salt, and black pepper.
6. Combine and knead the ingredients thoroughly.
7. Wrap a baking sheet in parchment paper.
8. Form the mixture into 20-25 centimeter-diameter balls and position them on the baking sheet.
9. Bake the patties at 250 degrees Celsius for approximately 45 to 50 minutes.

Butternut Squash With Chickpeas

2

Pinch of dill
  Pinch of all spice
  Pinch of cayenne pepper
1/7 tsp of sea salt

 250 oz. cooked chickpeas
2 1 section of a butternut squash
½ plum tomato
½ cup coconut milk
 2 cup water (add more water to make
thinner soup)

1. Add all the ingredients to a blender and blend to your desired consistency.
2. Add the blended ingredients
3. to a saucepan over a medium/high flame until it starts to boil or air bubbles rise.
4. Adjust it into low heat and cook for 60 minutes.

Asparagus In Formal Attire• Grated lemon
- Juice of 2 lemon
- Fresh thyme

- 24 stems of asparagus
- 16 springs of onions
- 4 tbsp of melted butter

DIRECTIONS :

1. In a steamer, cook the spring onion and asparagus for four mins, or until they are just soft enough to your liking.

2. Then, to prepare a dressing, combine the lemon rind, avocado butter, juice, and thyme.

3. If the lemon flavor is overpowering, try adding a few drops of cold-pressed extra virgin olive oil.

4. Spring onion and asparagus may now be dressed in a stylish stack.

Non-Dairy Apple Parfait

Ingredients:

2 cup chopped apple
1/2 cup rolled gluten-free oats, uncooked
2 tbsp. hemp seeds
1 cup soaked raw cashews 1 cup unsweetened almond or coconut milk
1 tsp. vanilla

DIRECTIONS:

In a blender, combine cashews, almond milk, and vanilla until smooth. In a small bowl, layer the following ingredients: a generous spoon of cashew cream, a quarter-cup of almonds, a sprinkle of oat and hemp seeds, and enjou!

Delicious Vegetable Potato Taler

450 g frozen vegetables 200 g grated cheese
20 g parsley
Nutmeg to taste
Some black pepper
250 g peeled potatoes
200 g white bread
2 egg, size L

Preparation:

1. The potatoes are peeled and cut into tiny cubes.

2. Then, permit the vegetables to thaw. Simply slice fresh produce into small segments.

3. Now bring a pot of water to a simmer and add the peeled potatoes for approximately 1-5 minutes. Reduce the heat until the water no longer boils.

4. Now add the vegetables and cook for another 1-5 minutes.

5. Then, drain the potatoes and vegetables, place them in a blender, and puree until smooth.

6. Cube the bread and mince the parsley to a fine consistency.

7. Place both ingredients in a larger basin with the egg and cheese.

41

8. Now combine all of the ingredients and form 15-20 taler, depending on the desired dimensions.

9. Then, line a baking sheet with parchment paper and distribute the dough on it.

10. To faintly brown the thalers, preheat the oven to 150°C convection and bake them for about 20 minutes.

www.ingramcontent.com/pod-product-compliance
Lightning Source LLC
Chambersburg PA
CBHW060628030426
42337CB00018B/3255